Weight Loss Motivation Secrets

Michael Kelly

ISBN-13: 978-1533062260
ISBN-10: 1533062269

CONTENTS

Introduction...vii

What is Your Teachability Index?................................ 1

Secret #1: What is your WHY?..................................... 5

Secret #2: Focus on What You Want - Create
SMART Goals 7

Secret #3: Become the Person..................................... 13

Secret #4: Use the Power of Small Wins 15

Secret #5: Create Positive Rituals............................. 18

Secret #6: Make it Fun... 21

Secret #7: Commit with Accountability.................. 23

Secret #8: Weekly Review 26

The 4 Pillars of Weight Loss...................................... 28

Your Three Day "Small Wins" Plan 39

Decide to Take Control.. 41

Free Gift 42

About the Author 43

Personal Notes 44

Michael Kelly

Introduction

What if I told you there was some information that you could get that would change your life forever, because it would allow you to become the type of person you need to be to create the change you want to create? You see, change starts with the individual. You have to make the decision for yourself.

What if I then told you that first you have to pay $20 to get a 300 page book AND read it? But only 5% of people actually read a book after buying it, and it takes weeks for most people to read a book. And of those 5%, only a very small percentage take action and get positive results because they don't have a clear plan to get where they want to go.

See, people like to buy 300 page books because it makes them feel like they are getting their money's worth. But if you don't read more than a few pages or even crack it open, you won't get your money's worth. Even if you do, you may be wasting time sorting through fluff and stories that will not get you closer to your goal.

My Promise

I promise to give you "straight to the point" information that is easy to use, simple to implement, and most importantly... PRODUCES RESULTS!

The information in this book is about creating lasting change in your life. Diets and fads come and go. What you want is lasting change. I am going to give you the tips and tricks you need to become the person that produces those results.

What is Your Teachability Index?

Do you 'know it all?' Have you read every single diet book out there and tried everything? In other words, is your teachability index low?

Be teachable. Approach this book like a student fresh off the bus. If you've heard it all before, hear it again with a fresh mind. You might have missed something the first few times through.

Listen. Forget the fact that this e-book is short. Forget everything you know or think you know. Just give this book a chance. What can it hurt? You might invest 30 minutes of your time in yourself, and gain at least one great insight to make positive change in your life. You have nothing to lose. This quick read gives you all of the good and none of the fluff to get the positive results you're after and set you on the right path.

95% of all diets and weight loss programs DO work, for nearly all people. There are some exceptions because of different body types and other factors. However, for the most part they work. That doesn't mean they are all healthy for you, but you can lose weight if you follow the various systems out there.

That's where the problem lies. We try to follow systems without understanding how we should follow them. We humans only succeed when we commit to 'mastery.' That means doing things over and over again, every single day. This isn't always exciting, but it does work. The trick is to get small wins and gain momentum. We'll show you how.

If you take a minute to read some Amazon reviews on any weight loss book you'll find people saying things like "there's nothing new in this book".

If that's your attitude, you're in danger. That's the attitude of someone who will never have the body they desire for any significant length of time. Whenever I hear someone make that type of comment, I can't take them seriously. Because I know they are not interested in mastery. They aren't interested in the fundamentals. And the thing is, fundamentals are what works. How so?

John Wooden's Advice

"If you keep too busy learning the tricks of the trade, you may never learn the trade."

John Wooden is the most consistent winning coach in college basketball history. He won ten NCAA national championships in a 12-year period, including an unprecedented seven in a row. His way of coaching had his players practice the fundamentals beyond the point that boredom set in, so that when it came time to win under pressure, they could do it. The fundamentals are important.

Fads Come and Go

The problem is fundamentals are not sexy. That's why diet fads are so popular. We want the shiny new object and everything that goes with it.

There isn't much new in the world when it comes to weight loss plans. Most of the time it's a new spin on an old idea. A fad with a new name. And that doesn't help anyone in the long term. Marketers have figured out this a new way to sell stuff.

Many people are able to lose weight multiple times over many years, using many different weight loss plans and diet pills. A new fad diet shows up and people jump on it, lose weight, and then later gain it back because the "new" wore off. They didn't commit to mastery and changing their habits, attitudes, and lifestyle. You have to work on YOU on a deeper level in order to change.

Most people don't want to hear this. They want a "quick-fix" to solve their problems. But maybe the problem is the person's mindset. You see, the same thinking that got you into a problem must be changed in order to solve the problem.

Before You Go Any Further...

Go buy a simple notebook. This will be your "journal" for the entire process. Throughout this book there will be assignments for you to do. These are VERY important. You must put in the work and do your homework. *This is not optional.*

If you want the results, you must commit yourself to the actions. You can do this. The actions are simple, easy, and enlightening. You will be glad you did it!

Secret #1: What is your WHY?

Why do you want to lose weight? Before we get into the "how-to" section of this book, let's talk about your reasons. Your WHY is the most important aspect of this entire process. It will be the reason you keep going when you feel like giving up. Your WHY is your reason for doing this.

When you create a strong and compelling why, you will have the strength and commitment needed to push through the difficult times. What will get you excited to succeed? What will give you the drive and energy to push forward aggressively after what you want?

Use reasons that create emotion in you. Logic often fails us. Of course we know we need to eat better, exercise more, and live a healthier lifestyle, but do we always do what we know we need to do? No.

Examples:

- I want to be healthier so I can be a good example for my children.

- I want to lose weight so I can fit into old bathing suit.

- I want to get in better shape so I can live longer and see my kids grow up.

Without a strong and compelling WHY, you have no reason to do what you are doing. What's the point if you don't have a reason?

Assignment

Take out your journal and make a list of strong and compelling reasons WHY you want lose weight. Be sure to make your reasons something that is personal and emotional to you.

Set a timer for 10 minutes and write anything that comes to mind. Do not stop writing until the timer goes off. Write down anything and everything that comes to mind. The more reasons you can create, the more power you will have to make it happen.

After 10 minutes, choose 4-5 really strong reasons and put a star next to them. We will come back to them later on a future assignment.

Secret #2: Focus on What You Want - Create SMART Goals

What do you want your outcome to be? In a perfect world with no limitations, no possible chance of failure, what would your perfect outcome be? Most people don't allow themselves to dream like this. They never even entertain the thought.

How can you get to your destination if you have no clue what or where it is?

I see this so often. It's very typical of New Year's resolutions. The majority of people set resolutions that are vague and undefined. With such a broad goal, how do you know when you have completed it? How would you even know how to go about creating a plan for a broad goal? It's very difficult to hit a target if you don't know exactly where it is.

Here's the solution. What result do you want? Be specific. VERY specific. Let's create a SMART goal.

SMART goals are:

- SPECIFIC

- MEASURABLE

- ATTAINABLE

- RELEVANT

- TIME BOUND

Specific

What exactly do you want to accomplish. You must define exactly what you want. A well-defined goal creates a frame to work with.

Bad Examples:

- I want to lose weight. (How much weight?)

- I want to start exercising. (What type of exercise? How often?)

Good Examples:

- I want to lose 15 pounds.

- I want to exercise at least 3 days a week for a minimum of 30 minutes each day.

This is a good example because it specifies exactly how much weight you want to lose, but it still has room for improvement. Keep reading.

Measurable

In order for a goal to be measurable, you must be able to quantify it. Whatever you can measure, you can manage.

You can measure pounds, inches, time, quantities, reps, miles, etc. Just make sure your goal contains something that is quantifiable so you can measure it often. This is how you will measure your progress.

This also leaves no uncertainty. Either you hit your goal or you don't. There is no gray area.

Measure your progress often. It will show you the progress you've made.

Attainable

Set yourself up to win. You want to set a goal that is attainable. Start with small wins and build momentum (We will talk about small wins later in the book). Momentum builds confidence, and confidence leads to greater action.

Make sure your goal is attainable. You want to challenge yourself, but do not make it so ambitious that you cannot reach it. Start small and work your way up.

<u>Bad Example</u>:

- I want to run a marathon before the end of the month.

If you have never even ran a single mile, this goal is not attainable for most people. Start small and work your way up. You may start with one mile. In a few weeks, you may run a 5K. A few weeks later you might even be running a half-marathon. Set yourself up with a series of attainable steps toward a larger goal.

Relevant

Make your goal relevant to your life and lifestyle. Be true to yourself. Make sure this is something YOU want. If you create a goal that you don't want, I can almost guarantee you won't give it your all. Create a goal that is relative to your life and situation.

It's time to be a little selfish here. Set a goal that YOU want. Don't do it for anyone but yourself. If it's something you truly want, you will work hard to attain it.

Time bound

There must be a start and end date. This creates a sense of urgency. Without a deadline, a goal is merely a wish.

Think of any task you had to do that had a time bound deadline. For instance, did you ever wait until the last minute in high school to do a term paper? How did you muster up the strength to pull an all-nighter to write it? Simple. There was a deadline and consequences for not doing it.

Parkinson's Law states that the amount of time one has to perform a task is the exact amount of time it will take to complete it. In other words, the amount of time you allot to your goal, your task will swell to meet that deadline.

If you think it will take you one year to lose 10 pounds, then it probably will. But if you give yourself four weeks to lose the weight and set a deadline, you will more than likely find a way to make it happen. Deadlines create a sense of stress (in a good way). This can get you motivated to take action immediately.

Create Your Own Goals

Now it is time to create your own goal. Based on what you have learned about SMART goals, start thinking about the perfect goal for yourself.

Examples of bad goals:

- I want to lose some weight.

- I want to start exercising.

- I want to eat healthier.

<u>Examples of excellent SMART goals</u>:

- I will lose 15 pounds before December 31, 2016 by exercising for at least 3 days a week for 30 minutes each time.

- I will lose 3 inches off my waist and be able to fit into my old favorite jeans before May 1, 2016.

Assignment

Take out your journal and create a SMART goal. Make sure it is very specific, measurable, attainable, relevant, and time bound. Set yourself up for success!

Be sure to download the free companion guide with printable SMART Goal sheets.

<u>Bonus Boost</u>

Post your goal in a place where you will see it daily. This could be on your refrigerator, bathroom mirror, in your car, or on your desk. Read your goal aloud every day when you wake up and every night before bed. Imagine what it will feel like once you have achieved your goal.

Secret #3: Become the Person

What traits and characteristics would a person that completed this goal have? Think about it for a moment. What kind of person would it take to complete this goal?

Let's say your goal is to lose 20 pounds before May 1, 2016. What kind of person would it take to complete this goal? You would probably have to be:

- Disciplined
- Focused
- Goal-oriented
- Health conscious
- Confident

Assignment

Take the time to think about this. Identify the character traits you will need to move forward.

1. Make a list of the character traits you will need to become the person you aspire to be. Set a timer for 10 minutes and write EVERYTHING that comes to mind.

2. Pick the top five traits that you want to adopt and put a star by them.

3. How can you implement these traits in your life? For each trait you listed, come up with 2-3 ways you can start implementing these traits into your behavior.

Become the person! Act as if you are that person. For an added bonus, watch Amy Cuddy's TED Talk (Your Body Shapes Who You Are) that talks about body language and acting as if. Amy Cuddy explains how body language affects how others view us and how we view ourselves. "Faking it" or "acting as if" can actually help you become the person!

Secret #4: Use the Power of Small Wins

The concept of small wins is something that has changed my life completely. The Harvard Business Review has written extensively about small wins in relation to work life. However it's much more than that. Small wins have helped people become champion athletes, top salesmen, role models, and much more. Small wins are what build momentum every single day. It's important to use this concept in your daily life. The whole idea is to start your day in a positive way that sets your mood to be good. That puts you in the right state to succeed with your goals going forward.

Losing weight drives performance; in turn, good performance, which depends on consistent progress, enhances your ability to lose weight and maintain your progress. We call this the progress loop; it reveals the potential for self-reinforcing benefits.

Celebrate your wins. Any habit you want to reinforce, celebrate the behavior.

Keep up with your wins and progress. Here are a few ways to keep up with your small wins:

Journaling – Each day before you go to bed, write down your wins for the day. It does not matter how small they are. Acknowledge your progress and be proud of it. This momentum will subconsciously remind you that you are improving each day. Improvement builds momentum and creates a sense of higher self-esteem.

Mark the Calendar – Each day you make progress towards your goals, put a big red X on the calendar. Once you start a chain or a streak, you do not want to end it. Keep it going at all costs!

Charts – Use charts to keep up with your progress. I personally like to use a monthly chart to keep up with new habits and routines I am trying to implement. Studies show that relatively small habits take about 21 days to take hold. I use this monthly chart to keep up with my habit progress and ensure victory!

Download the free companion guide that includes printable small win charts. Please visit:

www.motivationsecrets.org/weightloss

Secret #5: Create Positive Rituals

Is it fair to say that if you're overweight, it's a symptom of your life being out of balance? I believe so. If you want to lose weight, more than likely you aren't totally happy with other aspects of your life. It might sound crazy, but this is a good thing. Because the REAL solution to losing weight will help you put your entire life back in balance! The things you've probably chased all these years to lose weight, like eating right and exercising, are just a small part of the solution. The real solution is working on yourself, your life, to become a better version of YOU.

Most people think that having a set routine is too rigid. That it stifles their creativity. However, studies show the opposite.

"Rituals provide a stable framework in which creative breakthroughs often occur... The limitations of conscious will and discipline are rooted in the fact that every demand on our self-control all draw on the same small easily depleted reservoir of energy."

– The Power of Full Engagement by Jim Loehr and Tony Schwartz

What type of rituals and daily routines do you need to set yourself up for success? Here's a few ideas to jump start your rituals:

1. Start the day with a glass of water.

2. Eat a healthy and nutritious breakfast.

3. Exercise for at least 30 minutes per day 3-5 days per week.

4. Take the stairs when there is an option.

5. Wake up early to do something positive for yourself.

6. Journal about your life and your progress

7. Read. Find a book that will have a positive influence on your life.

Assignment

Take out your journal and set a timer for 10 minutes. Make a list of everything you can think of that would be a great daily ritual for you to start implementing.

After you've created your list, put a star by your favorites. Start implementing some of these rituals into your day. You are sure to see an improvement all around by implementing even one of these new rituals! You can add these daily rituals to your daily small wins chart from the last section.

Secret #6: Make it Fun

One of the problems I've faced for years is sticking to an exercise program because I get bored. Then I discovered podcasts. I like to listen to podcasts, audio books, and music while walking or jogging in the morning. This is a perfect way to start the day with quiet, easy movements that get your body moving and energize you.

You could listen to your favorite music and dance like nobody is watching. Sing in the shower. Be silly and playful. Make your day fun. Start the day with something that puts you in a good mood.

Whatever you have to do to get that child-like sense of wonder, fun, and excitement back, do it!

Assignment

Get your journal out and make a list of at least 10 things you enjoy doing. It can be anything. Think of ways you can incorporate these things into your day and find ways to make them a part of your routines. Not only will this have a big effect on your mood, but it will also make you happier.

Secret #7: Commit with Accountability

Accountability is a very powerful tool. How many times have you started a diet or work-out plan and did not follow through? Why? Probably because you weren't held accountable.

You need to find someone that will hold you accountable. Not only that, but you are going to create an incentive that will make you be accountable! This is why it's best to find someone who is either going to keep you accountable, or won't let you off the hook.

Accountability can be used a number of ways. Here are three ways that work the best:

1. Positive reinforcement

2. Negative reinforcement

3. A contract

Positive reinforcement is considered "pull motivation." You are pulled toward something positive and good. This is the strongest kind of motivation because it gets stronger the closer you get to your goal. However, it's the hardest to kick start. It can be very simple. Maybe you'll treat yourself to a movie at the end of your three day goal, or a weekend trip at the end of your 30 day goal. Basically, it is something that rewards you for good behavior toward your goals.

Negative reinforcement is considered "push motivation." It can be very strong. It's based more on losing something or embarrassment. However, we will use it a little differently. You need to decide on a negative consequence for breaking your commitment.

For example, you could post your goal on social media, and ask friends and family to hold you accountable. You could agree to check in daily or weekly and post pictures. This way, you will feel a sense of obligation to get it done because you don't want to let everyone down.

A Contract seals the deal. We humans easily deceive ourselves, so in order to make sure we follow-through, it is best to write up a physical contract with all of the terms of the agreement and sign it. It's best to do this with someone who will honor the contract and not let you off if you try to make excuses.

If you really want to seal the deal, choose an amount of money that will make you feel uncomfortable to lose. Give that money to a friend, and tell them they can keep it if you do not honor your contract. I've used this several times to boost my performance and get things done! It works even better if you know the money will go towards something you disapprove of. It almost seems that humans are programmed to work harder not to lose something we already have rather than gain something of equal or greater value. Keep this in mind when choosing your accountability boosters!

If you can get an accountability partner who also has the same goal of losing weight for themselves, that can work great. However, make sure it is not somebody that will allow you to break the agreement together! You want to select someone that will push you, motivate you, and challenge you to be your best self.

Download the free companion guide to with printable contracts to help hold you accountable! Please visit:

www.motivationsecrets.org/weightloss

Secret #8: Weekly Review

You must measure your progress weekly. This is not optional. The reason for this is to know more about your progress. That way you can decide if you are moving in the right direction or not. When things are going wrong you have to options. Do things differently. Or do different things.

Measure your progress each week. Set a specific day each week that you look over the past few days and see how things went. This is a time to learn about your behavior.

I personally use Sunday to review my week and plan for the next week. During my review I look over my wins and reflect on my progress. This is a time to be honest. If you did not meet your standards, it is ok. Review what went wrong and make corrections to set yourself up for success in the next week.

Assignment

Use these four questions below to access and review yourself every seven days. It is very important to review your progress often so you can course correct along the way.

1. What were your results over the past 7 days?

2. What went right? What were your strengths?

3. What went wrong? How can you prevent this?

4. What are your future actions based on your review?

Download the free companion guide to print out your weekly review sheet. Please visit:

www.motivationsecrets.org/weightloss

The 4 Pillars of Weight Loss

In the first part of this book we have worked on the foundation of this process, YOU. Now we are going to move on to the four pillars of losing weight and form a plan.

Each person is different and will want to go about this in different ways to suit themselves. There is a fundamental foundation and basis of losing weight and being healthy. There are no quick-fix schemes that suddenly give you the body you want. The foundation starts with you and your choices.

There are tons of weight loss plan out there. Most of them do work, but it requires discipline and persistence to achieve success with them. It is up to you to decide which one would work for you. Losing weight and keeping a healthy body does not have to be difficult. I want to break down the four pillars of the process for you to understand and give you some tips for each. The four pillars of weight loss are:

- Diet
- Exercise
- Sleep
- Stress

Diet

Your diet is one of the most important aspects of weight loss and maintaining a healthy lifestyle. You must be conscious of what you eat. One of the reasons I had you start tracking behavior earlier in this book is to get used to this routine. You want to start tracking the foods you are eating.

There are lots of apps out there that allow you to do this. One of my favorites is MyFitnessPal. It is a free app that you can download and use on your smart phone. Simply tracking your food intake can make you more aware your daily habits. If those habits don't support your goals, change them for habits that do.

MyFitnessPal is great because you can quickly and easily log your meals and get an instant overall view of your calories, fats, proteins, and carbohydrates. It is one of the simplest ways to keep up with your nutrition.

Here are a few tips for your diet:

Start your day with a glass of water. You've been asleep for eight hours and your body is partially dehydrated. Quench your thirst with water and hydrate your body immediately when you wake up.

Replace sodas and coffee with water. Make it a habit to start drinking more water. You should be drinking at least half your body weight in ounces of water. For example, if you weigh 150 pounds, you should be drinking at least 75 ounces of water a day.

Eat a breakfast high in protein. Fuel your body for the day with a breakfast high in protein. You can make a smoothie or protein shake, have eggs, or a number of other high protein meals. A high protein breakfast will make you feel "full" and less likely to snack throughout the day.

Cut your sugar intake. The typical American diet has entirely too much sugar in it. Sugar has been linked to tooth decay, heart disease, and diabetes.

Eat more soluble fiber. This includes oats and oatmeal, legumes (beans, lentils, peas), barley, fruits and veggies.

Reduce or eliminate processed foods. Eat REAL food. If you aren't sure if it's real or not, just don't eat it. Processed foods are usually high in sugar, sodium, or fats.

Have a smoothie or protein shake for one of your meals. Smoothies are easy to make, taste wonderful, and there are unlimited combinations of fruits, vegetables, proteins, nuts, and more to mix and make them!

Eat plant based foods more often. Have a salad with your meal. Start introducing more vegetables into your diet.

There is no magic diet that works for everyone. Like I said earlier, most diets do work. It's the people that fail. If you are not disciplined and consistent, then you will fail most of the time. You must be committed to whatever diet you choose. You don't have to choose a diet that makes life unbearable. Choose something that is right for you.

Exercise

If you fail to use it, you will lose it.

Your body is a miraculous vessel you use daily. If you neglect to use it, it will inevitably begin to wither. You must stay active and exercise at least 3-5 times per week.

Here is the good news... You do not have to work out like you're competing for a body building competition. There are plenty of simple exercises and techniques you can use to get fit.

Get active. There are lots of programs out there for every type of person. You don't have to join a gym to work out. You can do it from the comfort of your own home. You don't have to use weights. You can do lots of other activities to be active.

Whether it's just walking around your block daily or going to the gym a few times a week, try different things to see what you like.

You will want to raise your heart rate for at least 20-30 minutes at least 3-5 times per week. (Note: consult with your doctor before choosing an exercise program).

If you don't like exercise, join a class at your local gym to make it a social event. There are lots of Zumba classes, dance classes, or other types of fun movement classes.

Use YouTube to find something that you can do at home. There are lots of exercise videos and trainings online.

Plenty of apps are available to download that give you specific work-outs to do. It does not matter where you are starting from either. There is something out there for every body type, every fitness level, and anyone looking to better their lives through fitness.

There are no excuses. You might not know what to do, but there are tons of resources out there that will be right for you. You just have to look. You are only one Google search away from the perfect fitness routine for your lifestyle.

Sleep

Here is something you do not hear often. Get more sleep. Your body needs rest. Sleep repairs your body and positively affects brain function.

Lack of sleep can cause depression, anxiety, decreased quality of life, increased appetite, increased risk of heart attack, increased risk of accidents, irritability, and more. Think of the last time you didn't get enough sleep. How did you feel? There is a reason you felt so awful. Your body is screaming at you to get more sleep.

Sleep deprivation is a very common problem in our fast-paced world. Sleep plays a very important role in your physical and mental health. Sleep is involved in repairing and healing your body. On-going sleep deprivation has been linked to obesity, high blood pressure, heart disease, diabetes, stroke, and more.

Sleep supports balanced hormone production in your body. Sleep also promotes healthy growth and development in your body. Your immune system relies on sleep. Lack of rest affects how your body deals with sickness.

Remember earlier in this book when I mentioned, what gets measured gets managed? Well... good news. There are lots of ways to manage and quantify your sleep. There are lots of apps, tips, and tricks to use to increase the quality of your sleep.

Tips to Improve Your Sleep

Create a sleep schedule and stick to it. Try to go to bed at the same time every night.

Create a bedtime ritual. Do the same things each night to wind down and get ready for bed. Do something that relaxes you and primes your body for sleep. Try something like reading, prayer, or meditating.

Avoid TVs and electronic screens. The blue light emitted from these devices tricks your brain into thinking it is time to be awake. The have negative effects on your sleep.

Make your bed comfortable. Your bedroom should be dark, cool, and quiet. You should only use your bed for sleeping and sex. Do not watch TV in your bedroom. Do not eat in bed. Make your bed a special and comfortable place. Have blankets and pillows that are very comfy and relaxing.

Get some black out curtains. This is one of my personal favorites. Make your bedroom completely dark for sleep. This will work wonders on your quality of sleep.

Exercise or physical activity. Daily physical activity can promote better sleep. Don't exercise too close to bedtime.

Food and drink that promotes better sleep. There are certain foods that will help you sleep better. Try foods like almonds, yogurt, milk, bananas, or poultry. The reason is because they contain tryptophan which makes you sleepy.

You can also try herbal teas such as chamomile, valerian, or passion flower tea.

Sleep Apps

There are lots of apps out there that allow you to track your sleep and even offer soothing music to help your sleep.

Jawbone Up – I've used this app for years. You can keep track of your sleep and the amount of time you were in deep sleep or light sleep. It also keeps up with how many times you woke up and for how long. It requires you buy the activity tracker wristband, but it is well worth the money. You can also track your physical activity during the day, nutrition, and more.

Sleep Cycle – You can use your phone to track your sleep. While you sleep, Sleep Cycle analyzes your sleep for depth and duration, and allows you to connect specific daily behaviors, like exercise before sleep, to poor sleep patterns. When it is time to wake up, it gently awakes you during your lightest sleep phase to prevent grogginess.

Relax Melodies – This sleep app aids in going to sleep with smooth sounds and melodies that are relaxing. You can use timers and alarms on this app.

Stress

Stress is ever growing in our fast-paced world today. We all have stress. Stress affects your body, thoughts, behaviors, and feelings. Stress that is not resolved can have negative impacts on your overall health and your loved ones. How you handle the stress is what counts. Take some time to think about how you handle stressful situations.

Stress also affects our health. It can cause headaches, chest pains, upset stomach, high blood pressure, and sleep problems. Stress can be real or perceived. It can be created in the mind from things that are not even real.

Next time you are feeling stressed, stop and think about it. Where do you feel the stress in your body? What does it feel like? Being more aware of the stress itself can have a positive effect on reducing it. In order to solve a problem, you must know where the problem stems from.

Here's a few tips and tricks for dealing with stress:

Meditation

If you are anxious, tense, or worried from stress, consider trying meditation. You can spend only a few minutes a day to reduce the stress and restore a calmer sense of mind. Meditation is simple, effective, and freely available at any moment.

Here's the great thing... You don't have to

know how to meditate. You don't have to take expensive classes or find a special instructor. You can use apps on your smartphone that are free.

Here's a great start. Download the Headspace app on your smartphone and learn to relieve stress today.

Breathing

When you are tense and stressed, have you ever noticed your breathing pattern? Typically you will be taking shallow and short breaths. This manner of breathing has a major impact on the body. The primary role of breathing is to absorb oxygen in the body and to release carbon dioxide. When you are breathing shallow, you are not getting the full amount of oxygen in your body and not releasing the full amount of carbon dioxide.

Controlling your breathing can immediately melt stress away. Deciding to deliberately slow down and take deep breaths from your diaphragm can calm you down. Controlled breathing can create physiological changes in the body such as lowered blood pressure, increased feeling of calmness, increased physical energy, reduction of lactic acid, and reduce levels of stress hormones in the body.

Life is breath. Next time you get worked up or stressed, consciously take the time to slow down and control your breathing. Breathe deeply, inhale through your nose and exhale fully out your mouth. Do this for a count of ten breaths and watch the stress melt away.

There are lots of videos of breathing techniques online. Find one that works for you.

Your Three Day "Small Wins" Plan

Here's a jumpstart plan to create momentum for victory. Use this three day "small wins" plan to set yourself up for success. You can modify the plan any way you'd like to fit your goals and needs.

Small win #1: Start your day with quiet focus

Set up your day for success. Wake up 30-60 minutes early and invest this time in yourself. You can use this time to exercise, reflect on the day ahead, meditate, pray, go over your affirmations, or visualize your success. Use this time to invest in yourself.

Small win #2: Light exercise every single morning

Try to exercise early in the day. It will energize you for the rest of the day. Starting the day with a small win will make you feel great!

You can use this time to go for a light walk, stretch, do pushups/sit-ups, or do a work out video. Use this time to get your blood pumping and create a small win.

Small win #3: Eat a breakfast high in protein

Eat breakfast. It is the most important meal of the day. Try a healthy smoothie or protein shake. Mix in your favorite fruits or vegetables, yogurt, nuts, etc. Create something delicious and nutritious! Included in the free companion guide, there are over 25 delicious smoothie recipes.

Small win #4: Cut out the sodas. Drink water.

For the next three days, cut out all the sodas. Just drink water. Imagine it as fuel for your body. Water will keep your body hydrated, clean, and purified. Drink at least half your body weight in ounces of water.

Small win #5: Journal your daily wins.

Mark the calendar and journal about your day. Get your feelings and ideas out of your head and on paper. Write about the temptations and what you did to overcome them. Write about your victories and successes. Celebrate your small wins. Reward yourself for your victories!

Decide to Take Control

First of all, I want to congratulate you on making the decision to take control of your life. Life can be very hectic and feel overwhelming at times. Between family, work, and the demands of life, there seems to be little-to-no personal time for ourselves. I know the feeling.

By reading this book and doing the assignments, you have decided to be a better YOU. This is only the beginning. You have to be committed to mastery of yourself and your life. No one is going to make it happen but YOU. You are the captain of your ship and the master of your destiny.

If you haven't already, be sure to download your free companion guide to help you along the way. It is filled with printable charts, bonus tips, recipes, and more. It is designed to increase your success!

You can access it at:

www.motivationsecrets.org/weightloss

It has been an honor to share these tips with you. If you found this book to be helpful, share it with a friend. There's no greater gift than knowledge. Knowledge is power, but only when it is applied.

MAKE TODAY GREAT!

Free Gift

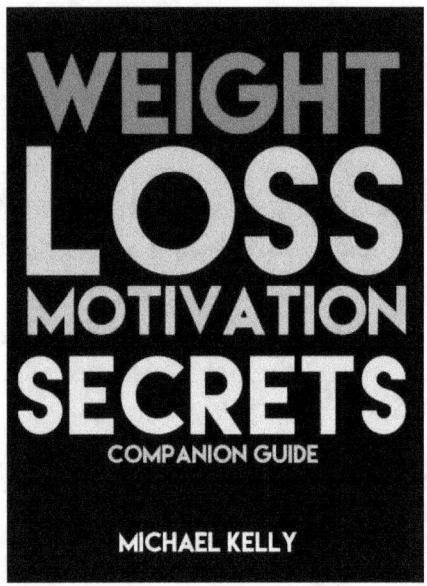

To download for free, please visit:

www.motivationsecrets.org/weightloss

Please visit the link above to instantly download your free weight loss motivation guide! It is a companion guide that goes along with this book. Inside you will find printable charts, recipes, and extra bonuses to help you along the way. Download it now!

About the Author

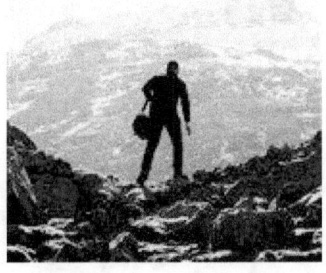

Michael Kelly is an author, self-development fanatic, and lover of life.

When Michael isn't writing you can find him hiking, biking, reading, or trying new things. He's a fun-loving guy that is open minded and cares deeply for others.

His life obsession is to find simple and easy ways to help others achieve their goals and live a better life. He dissects ways and techniques for improvement and explains them in an easy-to-understand way for the everyday person.

Personal Notes